INTRODUCTION TO HEART FAILURE

CAROL L. ALVIN RN, BSN

ALVIN & ASSOCIATES LEGAL NURSE CONSULTING

ISBN:0615789161
ISBN-13: 978-0615789163

1

Introduction to Heart Failure

Purpose

The purpose of this article is to provide you with a basic introductory understanding of heart failure.

Objectives

1. Define heart failure.
2. Name the two types of heart failure and define how they differ.
3. Name four precipitating causes of heart failure.
4. Name three medications used in heart failure and their purpose.
5. Name three diagnostic tests used in heart failure.

Heart disease is the leading cause of death in the United States. Heart failure is only one of the many entities that encompass heart disease. According to National Institute of Health 5.7 million people in the United States suffered from some form of heart failure in 2009 and of these 670,000 were first events. [1] Heart failure is not a single disease entity but "a complex clinical syndrome that can result from any cardiac disorder that impairs the ability of the ventricle to either fill properly or eject optimally. This syndrome results in a pathologic state in which the heart is unable to pump enough oxygenated blood to meet the metabolic needs of the body."[2] The inability of the ventricle to eject properly is systolic heart failure and the inability of the ventricle to fill properly is diastolic heart failure. These are two completely different entities and will be reviewed separately.

Etiology

It is important to understand the etiology of heart failure. Obviously patient teaching can decrease some of the risks associated with heart failure. The most common causes of heart failure are coronary artery disease, hypertension, valvular disease, and idiopathic. Less common causes include viral, dysrhythmias such as atrial fibrillation, endocrine, restrictive (amyloid, sarcoid, and hemochromatosis), and cardiotoxic substances (alcohol, cocaine).[3]

Clinical Presentation and Hemodynamics

Systolic dysfunction accounts for approximately two-thirds of all heart failure patients. Many of these patients may also have a diastolic component also. Systolic heart failure affects the forward flow of blood, thus decreasing the stroke volume. A normal ejection fraction (EF) is

---

[1] National Institute of Health. Morbidity and Mortality: 2012 Chart Book on Cardiovascular, Lung, and Blood Diseases. Page 19.

[2] Marzlin, Karen M. and Webner, Cynthia L. 2006. Cardiovascular Nursing: A Comprehensive Overview. Page 135-136.

[3] Davis, Leslie. 2004. Cardiovascular Nursing Secrets. Page 116.

55-70%. Typically the patient has a decreased EF <40% with a diagnosis of systolic heart failure.   For this reason the flow of blood to the organs of the body is affected. Often times symptoms of systolic heart failure will be related to specific organ systems. One of the first symptoms one encounters is **nausea, vomiting, and anorexia** due to decreased blood flow to the GI tract. The kidneys retain salt and water. The patient experiences muscle **fatigue, weakness, and exercise intolerance**. These are all symptoms of heart failure and specifically related to organ systems fed by the forward flow of blood pumped by the heart. Signs that the patient may have are **pallor, tachycardia, hypotension, and cool extremities**.

Diastolic dysfunction accounts for approximately one-third of all heart failure patients. There seems to be more women, especially older women being diagnosed with diastolic dysfunction. Although these patients are generally not as critically ill as those with systolic dysfunction they often fall through the cracks with their diagnosis being missed initially. Their symptoms are harder to manage. Diagnosis of diastolic dysfunction is not as straight forward as systolic dysfunction. Cardiac catheterization is the most reliable method for diagnosing diastolic dysfunction. Diastolic dysfunction has to do with the lack of compliance of the ventricles and this causes them to resist filling. This resistance to filling causes an overload on the lungs thus creating ones **shortness of breath, crackles, inability to sleep lying down symptoms**. These patients have a normal ejection fraction. Recommendations for treating diastolic dysfunction generally have to do with keeping the heart rate low and the blood pressure low.

Patients that have a combined systolic and diastolic dysfunction have a worse prognosis than those with isolated systolic or diastolic dysfunction.[4]

Diagnosing Heart Failure

First and foremost a medical history, assessment of risk factors, and physical assessment need to be performed. The following would then be more specific tests that might be ordered:

- **Lab work**: BNP (brain natriuretic peptide) can help in diagnosing heart failure
- **EKG**
- **Echocardiogram**: this is an important test for diagnosing and monitoring heart failure. It uses sound waves to produce an image of one's heart and helps to distinguish systolic heart failure from diastolic heart failure.
- **Ejection fraction**: this can be measured during an echocardiogram. Left ventricular ejection fraction (**LVEF**) is actually the measurement of how much blood that is being pumped out of the left ventricle of the heart with each contraction. It is used to help determine if the heart failure is systolic, diastolic, or mixed; so as to help guide treatment.
- **Stress test**: this test is done in order to see if the patient has coronary artery disease. The goal of the test is to assess how the patient's heart and blood vessel's respond to exertion.

---

[4] Marzlin, Karen M. and Webner, Cynthia L. 2006. Cardiovascular Nursing: A Comprehensive Overview. Page 137.

o **Coronary catheterization**: dye is injected via a catheter into the arteries of the heart to enable visualization to assess for any narrowing, coronary artery disease. A ventriculogram may also be done at this time which determines the strength of the left ventricle and can assess function of the heart valves.

Classifications of Heart Failure

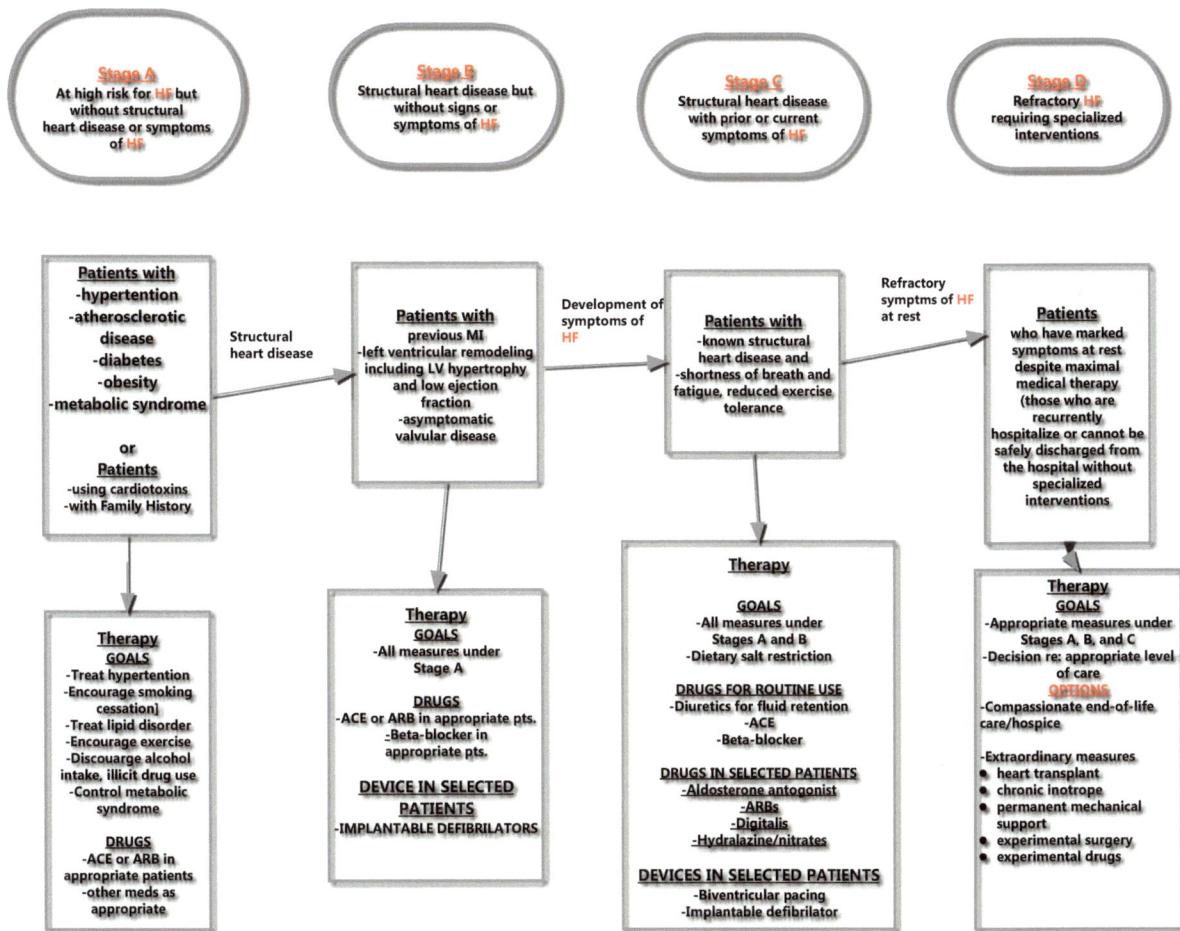

Figure 1. Stages in the Development of Heart Failure/Recommended Therapy by Stage. ACEI indicates angiotensin-converting enzyme inhibitors; ARB, angiotensin II receptor blocker; EF, ejection fraction; FHx CM, family history of cardiomyopathy; HF, heart failure; LVH, left ventricular hypertrophy; and MI, myocardial infarction.[5]

These stages of heart failure differ from the New York stages. The New York Stages of heart failure are stages I, II, III, and IV (mild, mild, moderate, and severe) and generally there is no movement back and forth between stages. Once a patient reaches stage IV that is where they stay. The patient's treatment, in the above classification system, is tied to these stages and the patient can flow back and forth between these stages. A patient adhering to treatment can go from level C back to level B.

---

[5] Jessup et al. March 2009. Circulation Journal of the American Heart Association. Page 1981.

Treatment Goals of Heart Failure

- Strict control of blood pressure
- Strict management of diabetes
- Aggressive control of risk factors

Pharmacological Management of Heart Failure

The following sections cover the different medications which are used in combination to manage heart failure.

- **ACE Inhibitors** (angiotensin-converting enzyme inhibitors): these medications vasodilate the blood vessels thus lowering the blood pressure and helping to decrease the workload on the heart. They act as an afterload reducer. Examples of these medications are lisinopril, enalapril, and captopril.
- **Angiotensin II receptor blockers:** there are a percentage of people that cannot tolerate ACE Inhibitor. An alternative for these people is the Angiotensin II receptor blockers. They produce the same effects as do the ACE Inhibitors. Examples of these medications are losartan and valsartan.
- **Beta blockers:** these medications slow the heart rate, decrease the blood pressure, and limit or reverse some of the damage to the heart. Decreasing the heart rate and blood pressure decreases the work load on the heart. Decreasing the heart rate allows for more filling time in people with diastolic dysfunction. Beta blockers also may reduce some of the abnormal arrhythmias associated with heart failure. Examples of these medications are carvedilol and metoprolol.
- **Diuretics:** heart failure is associated with fluid buildup in the body for various reasons. It is essential that any buildup of fluid is monitored and dealt with pharmacologically. Diuretics keep fluid from collecting in the body by increasing the rate of urination. Examples of commonly used diuretics are Lasix and bumex. It is important to remember that when taking a diuretic one will probably be losing potassium and magnesium so these will also need to be monitored and replaced.
- **Digoxin:** improves symptoms and exercise tolerance and is generally used on people that are symptomatic and already on the above three above medications. Digoxin has not been proven to affect long term mortality in patients.
- **Aldosterone antagonists:** these are potassium sparing diuretics and can actually raise the levels of potassium in the blood to dangerous levels. Modifying the diet of someone on an aldosterone antagonist is important. Examples of these medications include Aldactone and Inspra.

The above medications are only the medications that would be prescribed specifically to treat the heart failure. There would also be medications prescribed for risk management such as cholesterol lowering agents, diabetes control, and blood pressure control.

Contraindicated Medications in Patients with Heart Failure

Patients with any component of systolic heart failure should not take non-vasoselective calcium channel blockers. Examples of these would be Cardizem and verapamil.

Also NSAID medications should never be taken by any heart failure patient. NSAIDS indirectly cause vasoconstriction and decrease the effectiveness of diuretics. They also have a negative impact on the kidneys.

The Joint Commissions Core Measures for Heart Failure

The core measures were developed to help improve mortality and readmission rates for heart failure patients. Following are the Core Measures to be adhered to by all Joint Commission-accredited hospitals.

➢ Left ventricular function assessment
➢ ACE Inhibitor or ARB prescribed for left ventricular dysfunction at discharge or documentation as to reason that patient is unable to take medication
➢ Smoking cessation counseling for all smokers that have smoked within the last year
➢ Complete discharge instruction to include all 6 of the following:
   ❖ Weight monitoring
   ❖ Activity level
   ❖ Diet/fluid
   ❖ Worsening symptoms with specifics
   ❖ Medication reconciliation
   ❖ Follow up with physician

Missing any of these 6 discharge instructions is considered not doing any of them. Joint Commission monitors this activity when they do their evaluations of the hospitals. Hospitals are generally no longer receiving payment for patients' care when they are readmitted within 30 days or less of a prior heart failure admission.

Monitoring weight daily is very important. The writer of this CEU article developed this graph for her own use and found it very useful for her as well as sharing it with patients in the hospital. Stress to the patient that it is *imperative* to report whatever weight gain the physician decides on in the time period they specify.

DATE	WEIGHT	BLOOD PRESSURE		HR
		systolic	diastolic	
Jan. 31	150.6	117	73	61

Symptoms to report

The top five symptoms related to heart failure worsening are:

➢ Shortness of breath
➢ Decreased ability to exercise
➢ Orthopnea
➢ Profound fatigue
➢ Dizziness/lightheadedness[6]

Adherence to medication routines is imperative. Explaining the reasons for taking the medications to the patient is important. It gives them a reason for taking the medicine.

Activity

Obviously from the classifications listed above (A,B,C,and D system) there are four stages in the heart failure classification system. This system is an ebb and flow system. Activity is an important key to maintaining as high of level of functioning as possible.

➢ Reduces heart disease risk factors such as high blood pressure and being overweight
➢ Lower blood pressure
➢ Help increase energy levels
➢ Help reduce stress and anxiety
➢ Improve muscle tone and strength

Patients should always check with their physician first before following an exercise program but activity is encouraged. Warming up prior to aerobic exercise is important. One should wait 90 minutes after eating before doing any aerobic exercise. Warming down again after aerobic exercise is also important. Instruct the patient to always stop when noticing any symptoms such as chest pain, shortness of breath, or dizziness/lightheadedness.

---

[6] Albert, Nancy, Trochelman, Kathleen. , September 2010. American Journal of Critical Care. Vol. 19, No. 5, page 445.

Low Sodium Diet

➤ Decrease the sodium in the diet to at least 2 G per day. Some physicians ask patients to restrict their diets to 1.5 G per day. This is one of the most important ways to manage heart failure as it helps to decrease the fluid buildup in the body.

➤ Reading labels is important for sodium content.

➤ Include high fiber foods in the diet. Fiber helps move food along the digestive tract, may help reduce cholesterol, and helps control blood glucose levels. Also foods high in fiber include natural antioxidants which reduce the risk of cardiovascular disease.

➤ Carefully follow fluid management guidelines. These will vary depending on the severity of ones' heart failure.

Get With the Guidelines Heart Failure

These guidelines were developed by the American Heart Association to work for hospital teams, to ensure that they give evidence based quality care. Most hospitals that implement these guidelines realize measurable results. These are results not only seen in the lives of patients and families, but in satisfaction of caregivers, and in the financial health of participating hospitals.[7]

➤ The goal is to help each hospital that participates save lives by optimizing care for the heart failure patient. Progress toward that end is shown by studies showing reductions in mortality rates. Also fewer recurring events are seen.[8]

➤ Teams that use Get With the Guidelines have access to patient-specific guideline information and immediate access to clinical decision support through the American Heart Association's Patient Management Tool, which is an online, interactive assessment and reporting system. Using this system hospitals can track their program performance and zero in on areas that need improvement.[9]

Heart Failure Clinical Pathways

In the inpatient setting the important thing is that evidence based practice is put into place on a routine basis. The best way for this to happen is for there to be a map or pathway to follow. Thus came about the clinical pathways for the different disease processes. Below is an example of part of a clinical pathway with all of the requirements that you have previously learned in this article present (this pathway is simply an example and is not from any particular institution).

---

[7] American Heart Association. February 2012. "Get With the Guidelines." Retrieved March 19, 2012. (http://www.heart.org).

[8] American Heart Association. February 2012. "Get With the Guidelines." Retrieved March 19, 2012. (http://www.heart.org).

[9]American Heart Association. February 2012. "Get With the Guidelines." Retrieved March 19, 2012. (http://www.heart.org).

HEART FAILURE CLINICAL PATHWAY

Date			
Day	Admission – Day 1	Day 2	Day 3
Expected Outcomes	□ Pt. starting to diuresis □ Improved lung sounds □ O2 sat > 90%	□ Weight / edema down □ Labs within acceptable range □ Diurising continues □ Resp.status improves	□ Weight / edema down □ Labs within acceptable range □ Tolerating increased activity □ Resp.status improves
Nutrition	□ ___Gm Na+ diet Previous home restrictions	___Gm. Na+ diet Previous home restrictions	___Gm. Na+ diet Previous home restrictions
Test / Treatments	Foley needed? BMP BNP CBC Dig level if on Dig HgA1C if diabetes Lipid Profile TSH PT if on Coumadin CXR EKG ECHO_____% date_____ **Accurate I&O documented**	May d/c foley if present and diuresing decreased BMP ECHO_____% **Accurate I&O documented and weights recorded**	BMP **Accurate I&O documented and weights recorded**
Medications	Saline lock **ACE Inhibitor / ARB** (if not, why not?) Anticoagulant **Beta Blocker** (if not, why not?) Bowel protocol Digoxin po / IV Lasix IV KCl • Reconcile home medications with physician		
Activity	As per physician order: • Bedrest • Up with assistance • BRP • Up ad lib	Progress activity as tolerated	Patient tolerating increased activity? Order PT/OT if needed.
Physical Assessment Date:	Wt._____ Hot_____ Nursing assessments Dig level (if drawn) _____ K+_____ BUN/CR_____ Hgb_____ BNP_____ Pulse ox_____ Telemetry	Wt._____ Nursing assessments K+_____ BUN/CR_____ Hgb_____ BMP_____ Pulse ox_____ Telemetry	Wt._____ Nursing assessments K+_____ BUN/CR_____ Hgb_____ Pulse ox_____ Telemetry
	Admission – Day 1	Day 2	Day 3

Patient Education	Orient to patient pathway, unit and routines Assess readiness to learn Begin education if appropriate Initiate other consults if needed: <ul><li>Skin Care</li><li>Nutrition Services</li><li>Social Work (assistance with meds, no insurance)</li><li>PT/OT if needed</li></ul> Smoking Cessation documented (if applicable)	Confirm consults have seen patient Begin reviewing discharge instructions with patient: <ul><li>Need to weigh daily at the same time wearing the same amount of clothing</li><li>Low sodium diet</li><li>Medications</li><li>Signs / symptoms when to notify physician</li><li>Need to keep follow-up appointments</li><li>Activity restrictions</li></ul>	Continue to reinforce information: <ul><li>Need to weigh daily at the same time wearing the same amount of clothing</li><li>Low sodium diet</li><li>Medications</li><li>Signs / symptoms when to notify physician</li><li>Need to keep follow-up appointments</li><li>Activity restrictions</li></ul> Smoking Cessation documented (if applicable)
Discharge Planning	Patient's living situation: Alone Family Current with home care? SNF / ALF Plan for transportation home? _____	Care manager to address discharge needs.	Discharge needs addressed / finalized Home care_____ Rehab_____ SNF_____

In conclusion, *An Introduction to Heart Failure* has given you a glimpse into a very serious health issue in the United States. As stated at the beginning 5.7 million people in the United States suffer from heart failure. Let us get committed now to teach family members, friends, patients, and ourselves about the risk factors and work to help decrease these numbers. I touched on a variety of points from etiology, types of heart failure, tests for heart failure, medications for heart failure, The Joint Commissions Core Measures for heart failure, and I ended with a clinical pathway for heart failure. Heart failure really is a fascinating subject.

References
1. Albert, Nancy, Trochelman, Kathleen. September 2010. American Journal of Critical Care. Vol. 19, No. 5, page 445.
2. American Heart Association. February 2012. "Get With the Guidelines." Retrieved March 19, 2012. (http://www.heart.org).
3. Darovic, Gloria Oblouk. 2002. Hemodynamic Monitoring. Saunders. Pages 515-526.
4. Davis, Leslie. 2004. Cardiovascular Nursing Secrets. Page 116.
5. Dumitru, Iona MD, "Medscape Reference Drugs, Diseases, and Procedures: Heart Failure Medications", Jan 25, 2013
6. Marzlin, Karen M. and Webner, Cynthia L. 2006. Cardiovascular Nursing: A Comprehensive Overview. Page 135-136.
7. National Institute of Health. Morbidity and Mortality: 2012 Chart Book on Cardiovascular, Lung, and Blood Diseases. Page 19.

ABOUT THE AUTHOR

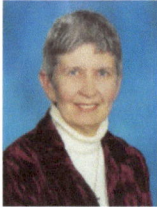

Carol spent all of her time in her 31 ½ years at the bedside where she had a passion for patient care but also a passion for teaching the nurses and residents that worked alongside of her. Carol Alvin received her diploma in nursing from Bethesda Hospital Nursing School in 1979 and went on to obtain her BSN at Xavier University in Cincinnati, OH in the mid 1980's. She spent the majority of her career at UC Health in Cincinnati with a focus on critical care including developing expertise in the surgical intensive care and coronary care, cardiovascular intensive care units and the post anesthesia care unit. She participated in the transition of the Coronary Care Unit to a Cardiovascular Intensive Care Unit which required intensive education. Carol was sent to the Cleveland Clinic for in-depth clinical experience with left ventricular devices (LVAD'S) and Heart Transplants and came back to Cincinnati, OH to be one of the 6 people to cross train the rest of the staff.

Carol received her Critical Care Certification (CCRN) in 1982 which she held throughout her bedside nursing career for a total of 30 years; and also received her Cardiac Medicine Certification (CMC) in 2010.

Carol has spent time teaching in-services to the PACU staff on neuro issues when she was a staff member in that unit. Carol presented in-services to the Critical Care Intern Program attendees. She was also an ACLS instructor. Carol also was a recipient of the University Hospital Hero Award in 2009.

Carol would like to dedicate this CEU project to her mentor Pat Iyer RN at www.patiyer.com. This project would never have seen the light of day without the selfless encouragement and motivating force she has brought to my life.

CE Test: Introduction to Heart Failure

1. The definition of heart failure is which one of the following?
    a. A decrease in the size of the lumen of the arterioles.
    b. Continuous ST elevation.
    c. A complex clinical syndrome that can result from any cardiac disorder that impairs the ability of the ventricle to either fill properly or eject optimally.
    d. Back up of fluid in the lungs.

2. Consider the classifications of heart failure. Which classification has structural heart disease but no signs or symptoms?
    a. A
    b. B
    c. C
    d. D

3. Which statement best describes the definition of Ejection Fraction?
    a. The amount of blood pumped out of the right atrium over 60 minutes.
    b. The measurement of how much blood is being pumped out of the ventricle with each contraction (can be left or right).
    c. The measurement of blood passively passed from the left atrium to the left ventricle.
    d. The amount of blood in the aorta after the heart empties.

4. Name the two types of heart failure.
    a. Sarcoid and amyloid.
    b. Systemic and central.
    c. Systolic and diastolic.
    d. Peripheral and central.

5. Name the diagnostic tests that should be done when diagnosing heart failure.
    a. Lab work—BNP
    b. EKG
    c. Echocardiogram
    d. Left Ejection Fraction Measured
    e. Stress Test
    f. Cardiac catheterization
    g. All of the above

6. Which of the medications below is the least important medication used in treating heart failure?

a. Ace Inhibitors
b. Beta blockers
c. Digoxin
d. Lasix
e. All of the above

7. Name four precipitating causes of heart failure.
   a. Coronary artery disease
   b. Hypertension
   c. Alcohol abuse
   d. Valvular disease
   e. Restrictive.
   f. All of the above.

8. Name three major symptoms of heart failure.
   a. Cough, headache, depression.
   b. Shortness of breath, swollen legs, GI symptoms.
   c. Decreased pulses, atrial fibrillation, headache.
   d. Tachycardia, hypertension, wide pulse pressure.

9. The Core Measures for Heart Failure were written by what agency?
   a. American Heart Association
   b. National Institute of Health
   c. Joint Commission
   d. AACN

10. Which of the following amounts of fluids would be a reasonable amount for a fluid restriction?
    a. 3000ml
    b. 2500ml
    c. 2000ml
    d. 500ml

Answer Key

1.c 2.b 3.b 4.c5. g6.c 7.f8.b 9.c10.c

COURSE EVALUATION

A=Agree   B=Neutral   C=Disagree

OBJECTIVES: After completing this course, I am able to
1. Discuss the types of heart failure and their differences.
2. Discuss medications used in the treatment of heart failure.
3. Name the core values identified in heart failure by the Joint Commission.
4. Discuss important issues in patient education in the area of heart failure.
5. Discuss the importance of a clinical pathway.
6. Discuss the types of tests used to diagnose heart failure.

COURSE CONTENT
7. The course materials were presented in a well-organized and clearly written manner.
8. The course expanded my knowledge and enhanced my skills related to the subject matter.
9. I intend to apply the knowledge and skills I've learned to my nursing practice. (Select the appropriate response below.)

A=YES   B=Unsure   C=NO   D=N/A

ATTESTATION
10. By submitting this answer sheet, I certify that I have read the course materials and personally completed the final examination based on the material presented. Mark "A" for Agree and "B" for Disagree.

Continuing Education Registration Form

Course Name: Introduction to Heart Failure

Participant Information: Please Print Clearly

This information will be used for your Completion Certificate. (Home address preferred.)

Name: _____

Street: _____

City, State, Zip _____

Phone: _____

RN___ LVN___ LPN___ Other title_____

License number: _____

Date of Completion for Certificate: _____

CEU Credits: Total number of contact hours for course: 3.0

Answers to Test Questions if applicable.

Participant has completed all course requirements: _____

Signature

*Please Note:

Taylor College will be issuing your Certificate of Completion for this course. "Provider is approved by the California Board of Registered Nursing, Provider Number CEP-3285, for the stated number of contact hours." This course is accepted for CE credit in ALL STATES. This course will also meet requirements for many national accrediting organizations. Please contact us or your National Board for confirmation. Fill in this form and return it, with a payment of $15.00 for your certificate.

Thank You for your participation.

Taylor College for Continuing Education 1-800-743-4006 (8-6 PT)

P.O. Box 93666 FAX:(323) 205-4390

Los Angeles, CA 90093-0666 Email: TaylorCEU@aol.com

  ___ mail certificate to you Email or FAX certificate to:

  _____

Please copy the above form to send to Taylor College along with proof of purchase of this article, or contact the author, Carol Alvin for a form at carol@alvinandassociateslnc.com

REFERENCE SECTION

Heart Failure Core Measure Set

Left ventricular function assessment

ACE Inhibitor or ARB prescribed for left ventricular dysfunction at discharge or documentation as to reason that patient is unable to take medication

Smoking cessation counseling for all smokers that have smoked within the last year

Complete discharge instruction to include all 6 of the following:

❖ Weight monitoring
❖ Activity level
❖ Diet/fluid
❖ Worsening symptoms with specifics
❖ Medication reconciliation
❖ Follow up with physician

MEDICATIONS FOR THE TREATMENT OF CHRONIC HEART FAILURE

- **Angiotensin-converting enzyme (ACE) inhibitors**. ACE inhibitors lower blood pressure, improve blood flow and decrease your heart's workload. These medications prevent the conversion of angiotensin I to angiotensin II, a potent vasoconstrictor.

  - **Captopril**
  - **Enalapril** (Vasotec)—helps to control blood pressure and proteinuria. Enalapril decreases the pulmonary-to-systemic flow ratio in the catheterization laboratory and increases systemic blood flow in patients with relatively low pulmonary vascular resistance. It has a favorable clinical effect when administered over a long period. It helps prevent potassium loss in distal tubules. The body conserves potassium; thus, less oral potassium supplementation is needed.[10]
  - **Lisinopril** (Prinivil, Zestril)—has been shown to decrease mortality after myocardial infarction.
  - **Ramipril** (Altace)—has been shown to decrease mortality in heart failure patients after myocardial infarction.
  - **Quinapril** (Accupril)

- **Angiotensin II (A-II) receptor blockers (ARB"S)**. These drugs provide several benefits of ACE inhibitors without the potential side effect of a persistent cough. These medications decrease afterload and prevent left ventricular remodeling. These medications can also be used as add-on therapy for patients that have refractory heart failure symptoms despite optimal medical management.

  - **Losartan** (Cozaar)—used in patients unable to tolerate ACE inhibitors. This medication has not been demonstrated to improve survival in heart failure patients.
  - **Valsartan** (Diovan)—used in patients unable to tolerate ACE inhibitors. This medication has been shown to be less likely to be associated with the side effect of coughing and angioedema. At target dose this medication has been shown to improve survival in patients with heart failure and decreased ejection fraction.
  - **Candesartan** (Atacand)-- be less likely to be associated with the side effect of coughing and angioedema. This medication has been shown to improve survival in patients with heart failure and decreased ejection fraction.

- **Beta blockers**: beta blockers slow the heart rate, lower blood pressure and lessen the risk of some abnormal heart rhythms. Beta blockers also reduce hospitalizations and the risk of sudden death; improve left ventricular function and exercise tolerance; and reduce heart failure functional class.

  - **Carvedilol** (Coreg)—beta blocker with alpha activity. This medication has moderate afterload reduction and slight preload reduction.
  - **Metoprolol** (Lopressor, Toprol XL)—beta blocker, beta 1 selective. Used in heart failure to reduce heart rate and blood pressure. This medication does not have intrinsic sympathomimetic activity.

- **Digoxin**. Also known as digitalis, digoxin increases the strength of heart contractions and tends to slow your heartbeat.

- **Diuretics**. Diuretics prevent fluid from collecting in your body and decrease fluid in your lungs, making breathing easier. Diuretics remain the standard of care for acute heart failure.

  - **Furosemide** (Lasix)—**Loop Diuretic**--increases the excretion of water and inhibits reabsorption of sodium and chloride in the ascending loop of Henle and the distal renal tubules.
  - **Torsemide** (Demadex)— **Loop Diuretic**--increases excretion of water, sodium, and chloride. It is essentially twice as potent as furosemide on a milligram basis.
  - **Bumetamide**— **Loop Diuretic**--increases excretion of water, sodium, and chloride. It is essentially four times as potent as furosemide on a milligram basis.
  - **Thiazide Diuretics**—in patients that do not respond to loop diuretics thiazide diuretics can be added 30 minutes prior to the dose of the loop diuretic. This inhibits reabsorption of sodium and chloride and also encourages excretion of potassium, bicarbonate, calcium, and uric acid. Patients that receive thiazide diuretics must be monitored closely for hypovolemia, hypokalemia, hyponatremia, and hypomagnesmia.
  - **Hydrochrlorothiazide** (Microzide)
  - **Chlorothiazide** (Diuril)
  - **Metolazone** (Zaroxolyn)—diuretic of the quinazoline class. Interferes with the renal tubular mechanism of electrolyte reabsorption. This medication is used most often in patients with impaired renal function.

The above medication information was obtained from Medscape from the following section:

Dumitru, Iona MD, " Medscape Reference Drugs, Diseases, and Procedures: Heart Failure Medications",   January 25, 2013

WEIGHT AND BLOOD PRESSURE FLOW CHART

DATE	WEIGHT	HR	SYST. BP	DIAST. BP	WATER INTAKE

AMERICAN HEART ASSOCIATION HEART FAILURE

CLASSIFICATION SYSTEM

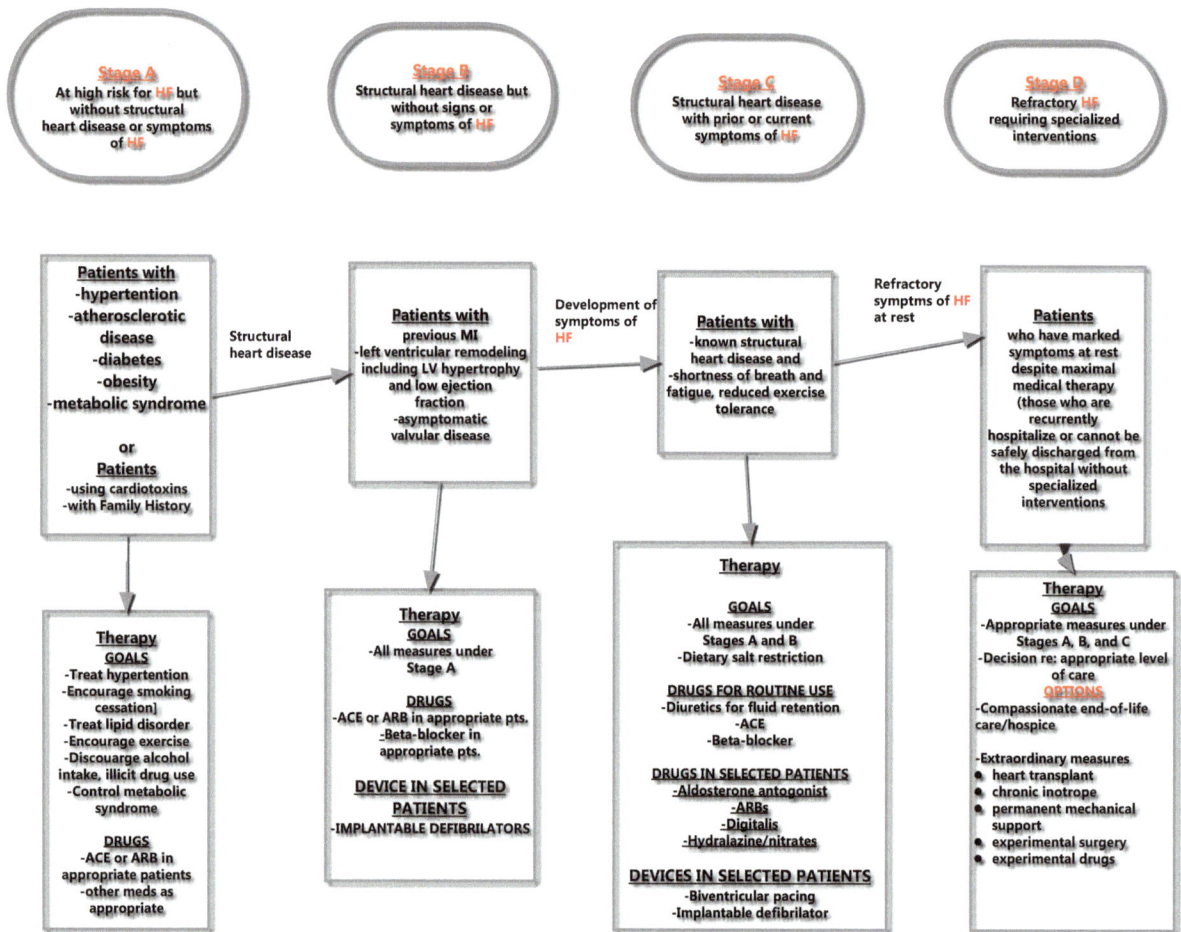

Stage A
At high risk for HF but without structural heart disease or symptoms of HF

Stage B
Structural heart disease but without signs or symptoms of HF

Stage C
Structural heart disease with prior or current symptoms of HF

Stage D
Refractory HF requiring specialized interventions

Patients with
-hypertention
-atherosclerotic disease
-diabetes
-obesity
-metabolic syndrome

or

Patients
-using cardiotoxins
-with Family History

Structural heart disease →

Patients with
previous MI
-left ventricular remodeling including LV hypertrophy and low ejection fraction
-asymptomatic valvular disease

Development of symptoms of HF →

Patients with
-known structural heart disease and
-shortness of breath and fatigue, reduced exercise tolerance

Refractory symptoms of HF at rest →

Patients
who have marked symptoms at rest despite maximal medical therapy (those who are recurrently hospitalize or cannot be safely discharged from the hospital without specialized interventions

Therapy
GOALS
-Treat hypertention
-Encourage smoking cessation]
-Treat lipid disorder
-Encourage exercise
-Discourage alcohol intake, illicit drug use
-Control metabolic syndrome

DRUGS
-ACE or ARB in appropriate patients
-other meds as appropriate

Therapy
GOALS
-All measures under Stage A

DRUGS
-ACE or ARB in appropriate pts.
-Beta-blocker in appropriate pts.

DEVICE IN SELECTED PATIENTS
-IMPLANTABLE DEFIBRILATORS

Therapy

GOALS
-All measures under Stages A and B
-Dietary salt restriction

DRUGS FOR ROUTINE USE
-Diuretics for fluid retention
-ACE
-Beta-blocker

DRUGS IN SELECTED PATIENTS
-Aldosterone antagonist
-ARBs
-Digitalis
-Hydralazine/nitrates

DEVICES IN SELECTED PATIENTS
-Biventricular pacing
-Implantable defibrilator

Therapy
GOALS
-Appropriate measures under Stages A, B, and C
-Decision re: appropriate level of care
OPTIONS
-Compassionate end-of-life care/hospice

-Extraordinary measures
• heart transplant
• chronic inotrope
• permanent mechanical support
• experimental surgery
• experimental drugs

21

NEW YORK HEART ASSOCIATION CLASSIFICATION SYSTEM FOR HEART FAILURE (obtained from the Heart Failure Society of America's Website)

CLASS I (Mild)	No limitation of physical activity. Ordinary physical activity does not cause any untoward symptoms.
CLASS II (Mild)	Slight limitation of physical activity. Comfortable at rest, but ordinary physical activity causes fatigue, palpitations, and dyspnea.
CLASS III (Moderate)	Marked limitation of physical activity. Comfortable at rest but less than ordinary activity causes fatigue, palpitations, and dyspnea.
CLASS IV (Severe)	Unable to carry out any physical activity without significant discomfort; symptoms of cardiac insufficiency at rest.

I Have a Passion for Helping Save Animals in Need. I have Six Rescue Dogs myself: JD, Shadow, Gracie, Manx, Bailey, and Peyton.

I lost a Very Special Friend on December 27…..Shasta……

I adopted her from Best Friends Animal Sanctuary in Kanab, UT 4 years prior when she was approximately 9 years old. She truly changed my life.

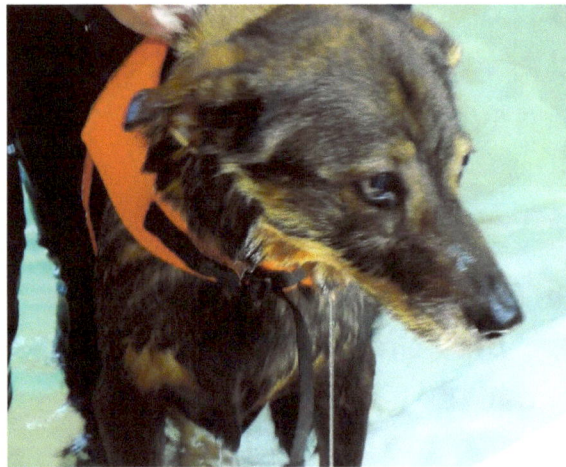

In Memory of Shasta I am donating 20% of the proceeds brought in by the sale of this book to

Pets in Need of Greater Cincinnati

Their "mission is to provide basic veterinary care for the owned companion animals of lower-income families in the Greater Cincinnati region, with particular emphasis on outlying areas where access to such care is limited.
They advocate and facilitate spay/neuter as an integral part of pet heath, as well as a means of controlling pet over-population in the region, and will assist in situations where individuals are overwhelmed by the needs of the animals in their care in order to prevent neglect, abuse and/or abandonment of these animals."

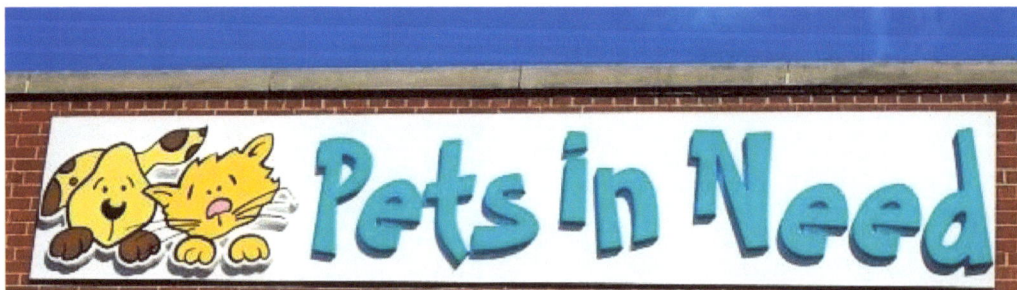